GIGA-ENERGY
HIGH ENERGY FOOD, HIGH ENERGY SNACKS

S. K. PILGRIM

TO MY WIFE AND MY SON, THIS BOOK IS FOR YOU.

GIGA-ENERGY
HIGH ENERGY FOOD, HIGH ENERGY SNACKS

Table of Contents

INTRODUCTION

Like every machine needs fuel to function and without the fuel, they are of no use and cannot perform, be it a car, bike, or airplane, the fuel type might change but they need one to function. The human body is the most complex machine on earth, and it needs fuel to convert it into energy and so that our body works properly daily. Well, the human body's fuel is food and it needs different types of fuel in the form of different food to function healthily. The human body is the most complex machine because every part it contains (muscles, brain, heart, liver) needs energy, different foods provide different types of energy which are helpful in the functioning of different parts and organs.

There are generally three types of energy sources which are fats, proteins, and carbohydrates. Energy from fats is the slowest source of energy and the body can store any excess energy into the body fats. Proteins are very important macronutrients of our body, they are used to build or repair tissues, muscles, bones and they can also be the source of energy but unlike fats and carbohydrates, our body does not store the excessive proteins. Carbohydrates are the quickest source of energy, once consumed they are immediately broken down into sugars (glucose, fructose, galactose) to be used for the tasks. The unused sugars will be converted into glycogen and stored in the muscles and liver to be used in the future.

The coming up chapters will explain in detail what types of food are the best energy sources, what food to have to boost energy instantly, what types of energy food are ideal while losing weight, what food keeps the energy up for a longer time, and much more coming your way.

Chapter 1

INSTANT ENERGY BOOSTERS

In everyday routine life, we come across a situation where we need an instant energy booster to cope up with our tasks. It includes every one of us, instant energy is required to the ones tired in the office but still have to finish a lot of work, to the ones going to work out, and even to teenagers who are stressed for their exams or got tired from long classes in the school. We all need the energy boosters to go through that tired phase. Here are some food that will provide instant energy:

Banana

Banana is an excellent source of instant energy, it's rich in potassium, fiber, vitamin B-6 and it provides instant and sustained energy to our body. It's a great source of instant energy and can be taken easily even in your offices as snacks, before hitting the gym or anywhere to give you that needed energy boost. Bananas can be used with much other food to have the maximum energy and a delicious taste out of it. Banana with peanut butter would make a very high protein and energy-boosting recipe. Spread the peanut butter onto a white bread or on brownies and slice the banana onto it and you are good to go.

A milkshake of bananas is also a popular shake to provide a lot of energy, especially just before you start your workout. Bananas can also go with oats, which gives a sweet touch to your healthy breakfast. Milk, oats, and banana would make a perfect combination.

Oats

Oats are full of fiber, vitamin B, iron, and provide an instant energy boost. Oats can be eaten raw or in the form of porridge, in both ways, it's a great source of instant energy as it takes no time to prepare them or make them ready to eat. Oats are generally considered to be only breakfast food but actually, it can be eaten in lunch and dinner when added with other food items. Add chocolates and milk to your oats which makes a perfect afternoon snack. Add some fruits and Greek yogurt to raw oats to meet your late-night cravings.

Apple

Apple is one of the best snacks to boost your energy levels, the best time to have an apple is in the morning, have it with your breakfast and kick start your day full of energy. Apples are full of fiber and sugars which help in keeping up the energy levels. There are plenty of different ways in which apples can be eaten and some might look odd, but they are very delicious. For example, apple and peanut butter stacks: Slice an apple in a few layers and spread peanut butter on them, combine two slices containing peanut butter with them and that will make a delicious apple peanut butter sandwich. You can also make dry apple chips and use them as snacks at any time. It can also be used in the fruit salads; without apple the salad would be incomplete.

Yogurt

Yogurt contains sugars like glucose and galactose, and they convert to energy immediately hence providing immediate energy boost after having a cup of yogurt. You can have it raw or with fruits to add in more nutrients and a great taste to it. Yogurt is such a magical food that can blend-in with plenty of other food to enhance the nutrients and the taste as well. Yogurt could be a great addition in your vegetable salad, blend yogurt with mint and have it with French fries to have a creamy touch instead of using tomato ketchup with them. It can be used in many cooking recipes, such as chicken curries, vegetable curries, and lentils. Yogurt is ideal to use as a side item with your grilled meats.

Sweet Potato

Sweet potato is rich in fiber and is loaded with carbohydrates, which means our body breaks those carbohydrates into sugars immediately and that is why they are one of the efficient sources of energy. Sweet potatoes are also full of vitamin A and along with energy production they aid in good health as well. Sweet potatoes are a perfect addition to your salads. Boil them and add them in your vegetable salad, they are also delicious when eaten alone or with some sauce as well. They can be added to noodles as well to make your meal more filling.

Chapter 2

FOOD TO KEEP THE ENERGY LEVELS UP FOR A LONGER TIME

To get sustainable energy every day through a daily diet is very important, energy from instant energy boosters will not last long and if you have a whole hectic day ahead of you then you need something which will keep your energy levels up for a longer time.

To overcome this problem, we must consume a diet that provides sustained energy that will last the whole day. Carbohydrates and sugary food are tempting and give an instant boost but they do not last long when it comes to energy, instead of these or having another cup of coffee you should add more food to the diet which is rich in proteins. Our body takes some time to break down the proteins and they remain in our body for a longer time and keep fueling with non-stop energy. Given below is the list of food which provides sustained energy: Stiehl, C. (2020, April 02)

Salmon

Salmon is full of nutrients and it has plenty of health benefits, it is loaded with vitamin B12 and it boosts the energy, which will last longer and its nutritional elements are the natural resources to fight against the fatigue. Salmon also contains natural vitamin D, which also keeps you energized. So, if you are not out there in the sunlight, don't worry your vitamin D needs will be fulfilled by having salmon. It could be a great recipe for your lunch to keep your afternoon energetic.

There are hundreds of recipes to cook salmon and have it made favorable in different ways. You can have it with boiled veggies such as broccoli, a combination of both will make full of nutrients and proteins recipe. Salmon with spinach again is a powerful combination. Barbequed salmon slices can also be used in different types of salads. Slices of salmon can be used in homemade burgers to give you a high protein dose. Smoked salmon along with the boiled eggs is a protein-packed delicious recipe to have at lunchtime.

Chickpeas

Chickpeas could be used in many ways and they are used in many dishes. But if we are talking about energy that holds us up for some time, then roasted chickpeas might be the best option. If you skipped your breakfast, have a cup of roasted chickpeas and they will hold you for your next meal and in the meantime, you will not feel any less energetic.

Boiled chickpeas can be added to different kinds of salads, they are stomach filling and can satisfy the irregular cravings at any time.

Avocado

Although avocado contains fiber as well, our body digests them at a slower pace than the simple carbohydrates, which provides more sustainable energy and that is why avocado is here in our list. Avocado and honey juice is full of nutrients, filling, and amazingly delicious as well. Avocado is not very sweet when eaten alone, you can add some yogurt or cream to make it creamy and tasty. Think out of the box and try avocado with scrambled eggs for a new healthy and tasty recipe. Avocado can also be combined with bananas, pineapple, or berries

Dark Chocolate

Instead of normal sugary chocolates, go for dark ones. Normal sugary chocolates contain more sugar content and break down immediately when consumed. Choose dark chocolate especially which contains 80% or more cocoa, it will not only provide you an instant boost but also, you will also feel good the whole day. You can also add dark chocolate to your tea, milk, or coffee for a rich taste.

Eggs

Eggs are almost everyone's favorite when it comes to breakfast, they are filling and easy to make. It hardly takes 5 to 10 minutes to get your breakfast ready with eggs. Eggs are loaded with proteins that provide long-lasting energy for your whole day. The amino acids in the eggs are known for stimulating the production of energy, they break down the fats to boost the energy levels. Eggs are also rich with vitamin B's, which helps the enzymes to breakdown the food to provide more energy to our body.

Chapter 3

PLANT-BASED ENERGY FOOD

There are plenty of options for food that we can take and fulfill our daily needs of energy. But what if you are a vegan or want to choose healthier choices? What options are left to boost your energy levels without breaking the diet? Daily energy needs must be met as it contributes to the overall health. Well! Don't worry about it as the following list of food will be enough to meet your energy needs.

Coconut

The coconut oil is a good source of energy. It's perfect for people who get tired quickly. Consuming coconut oil provides sustainable energy which will last longer. The oil can also be used in cooking. It contains fat and saturated fats and does not have sugars. It increases (HDL) good cholesterol levels as well.

Hummus

Choosing plant-based diet and finding a high protein energy source is sometimes difficult and you run out of options. Hummus is low in calorie count, low in sugars, and in fats as well, but it's rich in proteins hence fulfills the energy needs. It could be a great snack, as it can be used in many ways by adding other food to it as well. It can be eaten with bread and with vegetables and can be added as a side or appetizer along with your main course.

Lentils

Lentils are an excellent source of proteins and other nutrients for plant-based diets. Lentils are one of the best sources of iron for you. Lentils contain complex carbohydrates and provide slow-burning energy and keep you away from fatigue.

Brown Rice

Brown rice is a great source of energy and it is also highly nutritional grain. Brown rice is rich in manganese which produces energy from proteins. The energy will be produced steadily and will be consumed in the whole day without crashing.

Pecans

Pecans are a great source of manganese, copper, vitamins, and minerals including vitamin E, A, calcium, potassium, and zinc. The use of pecans provides sustainable energy to our body. Along with boosting energy, they contain monounsaturated fats which are healthy for the heart, they improve digestion, they are anti-inflammatory, and have anti-aging properties. Pecans can be eaten raw, roasted, and used in many different desserts and salads.

Chapter 4

ENERGY FROM NUTS AND SEEDS

Nuts and seeds are high in protein, fiber, and necessary nutrients and they have plenty of health benefits. Along with their great health benefits, they are also one of the finest sources of energy that you can get.

Nuts can also be taken with many foods as well; they make a great combination especially with sweet dishes. Following is the list of the nuts and seeds which could also work as an energy booster: (Rise To It, & *, N. (2015, March 12)

Walnuts

Walnuts could be your energy booster snack; they are a great source of OMEGA-3 fatty acids and they can provide a boost in your energy. Along with that, they contain essential proteins that provide amino acids and they have great health benefits overall and especially for your heart's health.

Pumpkin Seeds

Pumpkin seeds are fully loaded with minerals and many nutritional values. The amount of iron, manganese, phosphorus, copper, and zinc in them made them a pretty good source of sustainable energy. Additionally, they are good for our brain's health, and they have anti-inflammatory properties.

Almonds

Every one of us knows how beneficial almonds are for our overall health. Their richness in proteins made them a great source of energy. A handful of almonds daily could keep the energy levels up the whole day. The use of almonds also fights against heart diseases as well.

Chia Seeds

Like walnuts, chia seeds are also rich in OMEGA-3 fatty acids and rich in proteins. The protein becomes the main source of energy. Chia seeds could be used with a glass of water or to give it some flavorsome fruit juice could also be added. The use of chia seeds also stabilizes the blood sugar levels.

Pistachios

Pistachios are full of fiber, proteins, and minerals. Pistachios are very good to keep your metabolism on a fast track and boost the energy levels. They are rich in vitamin B6, which helps the body to use and store the energy produced from proteins and carbs.

Cashew

Cashews are loaded with proteins, magnesium, iron, and vitamin B-6. They are an excellent source of energy. You can eat them as a snack instead of having any of the caffeinated drinks like coffee. Magnesium deficiency is linked to fatigue, by eating this nut IT can augment magnesium deficiency. Cashews help the body to break the sugars in the body to produce more energy.

Chapter 5

ENERGY FROM JUICES AND SMOOTHIES

We have made caffeinated drinks a routine in our lives now. Coffee or tea at breakfast or in the afternoon with snacks. Yes, coffee might give an instant boost but why not replace it with something full of nutrients which will boost the energy as well. Juices and smoothies have great health benefits and they could be the source of energy as well. The below list will cover the juices and combination of smoothies which are great at boosting energy levels.

Christina Manian, R. (2019, June 10)

Strawberry-Vanilla Yogurt Smoothie

This is a very refreshing combination that can be consumed in breakfast or a snack anytime in the day. Soy milk can also be added, and instead of strawberry other fruits can also be added as per your choice. Strawberries contain magnesium, phosphorus, iron, calcium, and protein as well, having this drink will boost the energy levels which will last long in the day.

Peanut Butter Banana Smoothie

If you have a hectic day ahead and want to survive that without getting tired, then this peanut butter banana smoothie is the perfect source of energy that you can prepare easily. You can mix banana peanut butter along with milk and your energy booster is ready. The drink will provide a huge dose of protein along with healthy fats, fiber, and carbohydrates which will enhance the energy levels.

Cucumber Spinach Juice

A combination of cucumber and spinach will make magic green juice which will be full of powerful vitamins and minerals, it also contains chlorophyll which is very good for the blood cells. Spinach is known for its energy-boosting properties and it will provide a long-lasting push of energy.

Beetroot, Apple Carrot Juice

Like green juice has its health benefits, this red juice also has its unique benefits, especially it's good for the heart's health. The beetroot is loaded with vitamin C, and the apple will provide the necessary fiber to get you going. According to Zelman, K. M. (2014, April 05). The Truth About Beet Juice, beetroot will improve blood flow and increase energy levels and stamina.

Chapter 6

DAILY EATING ROUTINE TO MAINTAIN ENERGY LEVELS

Morning fatigue is very common, especially if you do not have a schedule of eating and sleeping well. Morning fatigue could be linked to many factors like lack of sleep, but one of the main reasons is low energy levels. To feel energetic every day, one must amend the daily eating styles to get those energetic results. Healthy eating habits are very important to keep you active all day and for overall health benefits as well. A daily healthy eating style must include the following: Delaware, T. S. (n.d.)

Consume a variety of vegetables:

You can categorize them as green vegetables and red vegetables. Green can be kale, spinach, cabbage, leaf lettuce, and collard. The red vegetables can be beets, radish, tomatoes, red cabbage, etc.

Add fruits to your daily diet routine:

A small change to your daily eating routine could be very beneficial for your health, for example, eat fruit daily between meals or whenever you crave for a snack. It could be a banana, an apple, or an orange.

Eat whole-grain food:

Whole grain food like brown rice, buckwheat, oatmeal, whole wheat bread, and corn. Try to avoid processed and carbohydrate food.

Have dairy items:

Dairy products are healthy but try to have low-fat milk, yogurt, cheese, and cream.

Low-fat protein food:

You can get a good amount of proteins without getting fat by eating eggs, beans, seafood, lean meats, and nuts.

Use of cooking oil:

While cooking tries to use vegetable oil instead of solid fat oils. Olive oil is best for cooking.

Restrict your junk food intake:

Junk food is full of trans fats and high in sodium which causes hypertension obesity and kidney problems. It's better to exclude junk food from your diet or at least stop having it regularly.

Replace soft drinks with fresh juices:

Try to eliminate soft drinks from your daily diet plan, instead of soft drinks, have fresh juices for sustainable energy.

Eat at regular intervals

Do not eat a lot in a single meal, that will make you sleepy and dull. Add a snack meal between breakfast and lunch and a snack meal between lunch and dinner. What snacks you will have may depend on your fitness goals. It might be fruit salad, mix nuts, peanut butter, or even just an apple.

Chapter 7

ENERGY FOOD FOR FAST METABOLISM AND WEIGHT LOSS

If you are trying to reduce a few pounds, it is very important to first understand this whole mechanism behind reducing the weight. A fast metabolism is directly linked to weight loss, the faster the metabolism is more calorie you will burn. To keep your metabolism fast you must keep your energy levels high to support that kind of metabolism. For fast metabolism and losing weight, you should consume food that is rich in proteins and not in carbs.

Below are certain types of food that could help in kicking on your metabolism. Petre, A. (n.d.)

Food Rich in Proteins

High protein food such as meat, fish, eggs, nuts, and seeds help increase metabolism, which means your body will consume more energy to digest them.

These high protein foods increase the metabolism rate by 15% to 20% which is high as compared to the metabolism rate increase as a result of consuming carbs and fats. Protein-rich food support in keeping the muscle mass while reducing the unnecessary fat deposits.

Food Rich in Iron and Zinc

Iron and Zinc both are very important for our overall health, they are both very important to the functioning of the thyroid to produce hormones. Less intake of iron and zinc will result in producing fewer hormones by the thyroid and this can slow down the metabolic rate. Hence taking the iron and zinc-rich food are very important.

Chili Peppers

Chili peppers contain a compound called Capsaicin, which helps in increasing the metabolic rate by burning more calories. Chili peppers are good to increase the energy levels instantly and give your body the job to burn some calories with an increased metabolic rate.

Coconut Oil

Coconut oil is an ideal source of energy, especially when you are trying to increase the metabolic rate and reduce weight. You just have to replace other fats with coconut oil, and it will increase your metabolism and maintain the energy levels as well.

Seaweed

Seaweed is a great source of iodine, which is important for the production of thyroid-related hormones and the proper function of the thyroid gland. The thyroid gland produces many hormones, some of which are responsible for metabolism. Meeting your iodine requirements means keeping your metabolic rate high, which ultimately burns more calories.

Chapter 8

KICK START THE DAY WITH FULL OF ENERGY BREAKFAST

Breakfast is a very important meal of the day, and you should have something which is filling and energizing at the same time to start your day on a high note. Breakfast should be heavy and loaded with proteins and nutrients to help you in getting through the whole day without feeling tired. There are plenty of high protein breakfast options, you can check out some below-given breakfast ideas to make your morning energetic.

Peanut Butter and Fruits Wrap

Breakfast wraps are easy to make. Getting late for office or your college and university, wraps are time-savers and you can make them as much fulfilling as you like. Just spread the peanut butter on a loaf of whole-grain bread, add fruit on it, banana, apple and berries are all the ideal choices for this wrap and they are perfect to provide you the energy that you need to start your day.

Oats with Fruits and Nuts

Oats are considered to be a boring breakfast for many of us, but if we add some fruits and nuts to it, it will be a refreshing combination and will give energy which will last all morning.

Whole Grain Cereals

Whole grain cereals are very easy to be prepared and they are high in fiber and protein and low in sugar and carbs, which means it is an excellent source of energy. Additionally, you can add fruits and nuts to it as well to load it with more nutrients along with a great taste.

Avocado Toast

One of the simple and healthy breakfast can be made very easily with avocado and a whole grain bread toast. Prepare the toast and spread the mashed avocado over it and you will have your morning energy dose. Avocado is rich in fiber and complex carbohydrates, which are slow to digest hence provide sustainable energy. On a plus side, avocados contain antioxidants which help in building healthy skin, nails, and hairs and those for sure are essential benefits.

BONUS

LOW-CHOLESTEROL HIGH ENERGY FOOD

For a good and healthy body, everyone needs energy and necessary nutrients daily. However, some who unfortunately have high cholesterol problems and they just cannot intake everything for the sake of getting the energy. They have to choose from the food wisely and to keep their energy up and cholesterols at a controlled level. Many foods provide a boost in the energy levels and are not only low in cholesterol, but they help in reducing the bad cholesterol in our body. Follow the below list to know more about such food.

Food Rich in Unsaturated Fats

Saturated fats are directly linked to an increase of cholesterol, cutting down the saturated fats diet will help in lowering the cholesterol levels. Instead of that include unsaturated food to your diet to maintain your energy levels and it will help in lowering the cholesterol levels as well. Some unsaturated fat food includes:

-Sunflower oil, olive oil, corn, and oil from nuts. Add these oils in cooking or preparing your food, these will keep the cholesterol levels maintained

-Add avocado and raw nuts and seeds to your routine diet plan

-Eat oily fish more often; fish like trout, sardines, and mackerel are rich in OMEGA-3 and unsaturated fats which helps in reducing the cholesterol levels. You should intake fish 2 to 3 times a week ideally. All these foods are a great source of energy as well.

Adding More Fruits & Veggies and Cutting Fried Food Items from The Diet

Fruits and vegetables are full of vitamins and minerals and they help in preventing heart diseases and stroke. On the other hand, fried food items are bad news for your cholesterol and not at all good for the heart.

There are a variety of fruits and vegetables that will provide enough required energy and they are ideal to control cholesterol levels. Fruits and veggies are high in fiber as well which helps in reducing cholesterol levels. Pulses, peas, sweet potatoes, eggplant, strawberries, okra, broccoli, and apples are one of the perfect solutions for your high energy low-cholesterol diet.

Soy Food

Food made from soya beans is healthy, high in proteins, and low in saturated fats plus they contain vitamins and minerals.

LOW-SUGAR HIGH ENERGY FOOD

Many of us consume sugar in our daily routine diets much more than necessary, which eventually have bad impacts on our overall health. If you are planning to cut those sugar intakes and maintain a sugar-free healthy diet and at the same time you want to take high energy food to keep you going then go through the below mentioned few foods which are low in sugar and can provide a boost in energy as well.

Spinach

Spinach possesses high values of iron, magnesium, and potassium. Iron is very important to fuel oxygen in our blood which ultimately becomes the source of energy. Magnesium naturally is an energy-boosting agent and along with potassium, they help in maintaining the energy, nerves, and muscles of our body. While having spinach you do not have to worry about the sugar levels as spinach does not have sugars.

Green Tea

Green tea does not contain sugars or carbs, and it can boost energy as well due to the caffeine traces found in it. It can boost energy levels instantly. On a plus side, it contains vitamins A, D, C and in minerals, it contains Zinc and Chromium.

Whole Grain Food

It is no secret how beneficial whole-grain food is for our health. To avoid added sugars, you will have to cut all processed food and focus on whole-grain food. Whole grain food includes all the following brown rice, Oats, Buckwheat, Corns, and whole-wheat.

Water

Sometimes we concentrate on all the other food which we think is healthy for us and we forget the importance of water and its link to energy levels. Lack of water consumption leads to dehydration; dehydration causes low levels of energy. An average man must consume at least 3 to 4 liters of water and an average woman must consume 2.7 to 3.7 liters of water to keep the body hydrated.

Conclusion

"We become what we eat", many of us must have heard about it or read this popular sentence. It's true, even a Research at the University of Oxford has demonstrated that the diets that we have over time can change the composition of the genes. This ultimately concludes that it is very important what we eat to get the necessary proteins and nutrients to boost our energy, as it will impact our health in the long run.

What we eat eventually becomes a part of our cells over a certain period. Paying attention to what we eat is important but we all should have awareness of how a particular food will be processed. To have all the information about the whole mechanism is very important to plan your diets and decide what to eat or what not to eat.

To know which food will be a great source of energy and at the same time will be processed by our body without any other complications like indigestion is very important. Hence, it is pretty much concluded that sticking to a simple and natural diet is a better choice. Eating processed canned food or food with added sugars or added preservatives should be avoided. Restricting the junk and all those artificially flavored foods might be difficult at the start but once you will see the positive results on your health you will get motivated to follow a simple, natural, and healthy diet.

Thank you once again for purchasing this book, and hope that it will aid you to have "GIGA-ENERGY" in your daily activities!

References

(n.d.). Retrieved from
https://www.naturalbalancefoods.co.uk/community/fitness/vegan-foods-for-energy/

foods that provide instant energy to the body. (2019, August 15). Retrieved from https://timesofindia.indiatimes.com/life-style/food-news/10-foods-that-provide-instant-energy-to-the-body/photostory/70677150.cms

Christina Manian, R. (2019, June 10). Energy-Boosting Smoothies That Will Keep You Powered Up. Retrieved from https://www.tasteofhome.com/collection/energy-smoothie-recipes/

Delaware, T. S. (n.d.). Eating For Better Health. Retrieved from https://dhss.delaware.gov/dhss/dph/dpc/eatright.html

Energy Sources in Foods: Carbohydrates, Fat, and Protein. (n.d.). Retrieved from https://www.e-education.psu.edu/geog3/node/1196

Petre, A. (n.d.). Best Foods to Boost Your Metabolism. Retrieved from https://www.healthline.com/nutrition/metabolism-boosting-foods#section1

Rise To It, & *, N. (2015, March 12). Energy Boosting Nuts and Seeds. Retrieved from http://risetoit.co.za/energy-boosting-nuts-and-seeds/

Stiehl, C. (2020, April 02). 30 Foods That Give You All-Day Energy. Retrieved from https://www.eatthis.com/foods-all-day-energy/

Zancan, K. (2018, August 15). The Path Magazine. Retrieved from http://www.thepathmag.com/4-fresh-juices-early-morning-energy-boost/

Zelman, K. M. (2014, April 05). The Truth About Beet Juice.

Retrieved from https://www.webmd.com/food-recipes/features/truth-about-beetroot-juice

Printed in Great Britain
by Amazon